I0102724

Illustration contribution: Cara Mastin

Editorial contribution: Jason Jones

Printed in the United States of America

Published by AFCP publishing

Email: info@afcppub.com

Copyright © 2011 Courtnye Jackson

All rights reserved

ISBN: 0615500919

ISBN 13: 9780615500911

Thanks to my mom & dad who support me in all my many endeavors and who taught me that I can do or be anything my heart desires. Also to Jason who is always there when I need him.
I love you guys!

*Dedicated, not to Americas top model, but
to the natural girls right next door.
Dead Prez*

My (brief) Hair Story

From the time I was a young girl, until about age twenty-five I wanted someone else's hair. Growing up, I was endlessly teased in school about my short nappy hair. The harassment made me feel my hair was unattractive. I wanted long loose curls like the women I saw on television, that bounced and moved with the wind. Not the thick crown that God had blessed me with. Throughout the years I tortured my hair in an effort to convert it into something it was not. I covered it with weaves and wigs, left braids in for months at a time, relaxed, colored, texturized, over-processed, heat-damaged, and neglected my hair. After which I would cry and pout when my hair did not seem to grow!

Through many trials and after two failed attempts at sporting natural hair, I finally stopped listening to the naysayers that told me 'I didn't have the right texture of hair to go natural' or that 'I was prettier with straight hair' and learned that my hair was beautiful. In 2003 I started my nappy journey and never looked back! I now proudly rock my natural, nappy, thick curls for all the world to see!

From my experience, many people with afro-textured hair have bought into the myth that our hair is not accepted, professional or attractive. I believe that because of this thought process the act of 'going natural' is about much more than hair. It is the courage to challenge the accepted perceptions and views of beauty as well as a mental shift toward self-acceptance and love. Now when someone makes fun of my hair, I feel sorry for them and am proud of the fact that I no longer internalize their insecurities or buy into false standards of what makes me beautiful. We are all ever evolving, but I can undeniably say that I love my hair the way it is and yes, I may find someone else's hair pretty or attractive, but that in no way diminishes the God given crown on top of my own head!

Your Hair Story

Write your hair story and share it with someone that you feel needs encouragement

_____

_____

_____

_____

_____

_____

_____

_____

_____

_____

_____

_____

_____

_____

_____

_____

_____

_____

_____

_____

_____

_____

Can you remember a time when someone made you feel negatively about your hair? If it's still bothering you, how can you resolve it?

_____

_____

_____

_____

_____

_____

_____

_____

_____

Here are a couple of ways to help resolve the issue

- Tell the person how you feel, honesty is always the best policy in this case, especially if you have to see the person on a regular basis. Try not to keep feelings bottled up and in some cases the person may not know they hurt you

- If you don't want to approach the person or they aren't easily accessible, you can write them a letter without sending it, writing can be a great catharsis

- Whenever someone makes a negative comment, make two positive ones for yourself! Keep positivity cards with you

- Share your story with someone who will either understand or listen and promote your natural beauty

- If you have issues that continuously resurface and affect your daily life, seeing a specialist might be a good idea or you could try speaking to someone that you trust about the issue

How does your reaction change to what others think or say about your hair the longer you are natural and what does this say about your mental growth?

_____

_____

_____

_____

_____

_____

_____

_____

Having trouble deciding to go or stay natural? Here are a couple of things that may help you decide.

- Make a pro and con list
- Speak to someone who has been natural for years, talk to them about their journey
- Take a note from Nike and 'just do it'! Take the risk, try it out and see if you like it
- Speak to a professional about natural hair styles if you want to big chop or get a transition style that makes you comfortable

Getting to know your hair

Getting to know your hair, how it feels, reacts to products and its general texture is a huge part of good care. The cornerstone of hair health is based on the fact that you know what your hair feels like when it's healthy. Since there is so much information to be found about hair out there already, we have included very brief and simple outlines of some important facts to get you started. We have also included questions and notes sections to take along if you decide to seek the assistance of a qualified professional

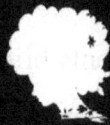

Sometimes getting your hair in optimal condition and growing it to the length you want can be frustrating, but remember the best part of a trip is the journey. Try to enjoy getting to know your hair! I still find myself combing forums and watching videos whenever I need inspiration and most importantly I write down my regimen. Keeping a written log and regimen is important when caring for your hair as it will keep you on track, make your hair a priority, and simplify the process. A regimen is especially important if you are recently natural.

Some tips that I've learned when getting to know your hair:

- Share what you know: it's always more fun when you share your story with others, exchange tips and give advice
- Listen to your hair: if you apply a product or do something that your hair does not agree with, it will tell you
- Ward off naysayers: negativity will only bring you down
- Don't listen to everyone: take what you think and know will work on your hair and go with that
- Trim your ends: A good trim will help ward off splits and breakage
- If you aren't able to solve it, see a professional

What key things have you learned about your hair?

_____

_____

_____

_____

_____

_____

_____

If you're not yet at your goal don't get frustrated, get inspired!

- Gather inspiration from natural hair care forums, blogs and videos, there are a plethora on the internet
- Get books specifically dedicated to hair care and keep notes
- Study your hair; learn how it responds to certain things like the weather, water, products, and manipulation.
- Make a vision board and post it somewhere that you can visualize it daily
- Get divine inspiration, pray it out
- Speak to your support team; get people in your corner who have been there and done that

When do you feel most inspired and positive about your hair?

_____

_____

_____

_____

_____

_____

_____

Positivity cards can be a great pick me up when you are feeling down. Create your own affirmations using note cards! Here are some suggestions to get you started:

I love my hair because…

I realize I am beautiful because…

My hair is perfect the way God created it!

What are some other affirmations?

_____

_____

_____

_____

_____

_____

_____

Away we grow!

Doing these simple things may enhance your hair retention & growth.
They may prove to be essential on your hair growth journey!

Practice patience, it's hair & if well maintained it will grow, but it will take time! Many times when we become impatient we take drastic measures to get the length we wish to attain such as glue in weaves or braids that are too tight. These actions can have detrimental effects to the growth that we have thus far.

Scalp Massages on a regular basis have been shown to increase blood & oxygen circulation to the scalp

Eating healthy & drinking plenty of water! Healthy body = healthy blood, which is essential to maintaining healthy locks!

Protective styling is needed to keep those ends from splitting and breaking off. It has been scientifically proven that hair health, strength and growth benefits from low manipulation.

Wrap it up! Wrap your hair before catching some z's. It's important to use something like silk or satin which doesn't cause unnecessary friction on the hair resulting in breakage, nor does it soak up moisture like some fabrics.

Be gentle with your hair, especially when it is wet, which is when hair is in one of it's most fragile states.

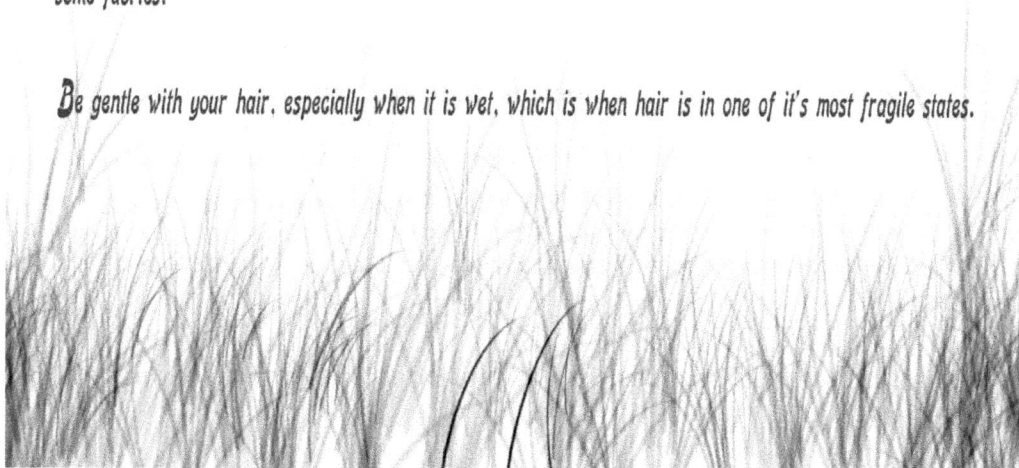

1. Scalp health

One of the most important aspects of hair health has nothing to do with the care of the actual strands, but your scalp! The scalp is where the follicles are found and this is where your hair shaft starts to grow. In most cases, healthy scalp equals healthy hair. Take note of how your scalp feels: Does it itch? Are there sores? Is it painful in one area?

Have someone, a professional or a close friend do a general scalp analysis. They should note if there are any,

- Flakes or dandruff
- Ectoparasites or bugs
- Alopecia or hair loss
- Build up, usually in the form of product, oil or sebum

Some general things you can do to ensure your scalp is healthy:

- Scalp massages not only feel good but they also serve to redistribute oils and increase circulation
- Check the ingredients on your products, because using products with harsh and dangerous chemicals can not only strip and damage your hair they are not great for the scalp either
- Take care of your body by eating well, drinking adequate amounts of water, and getting enough sleep
- Keep build-up at bay through regular clarification (making sure not to over clarify) and cleansing of the scalp
- Try applying chemicals, conditioners and other products to the shaft of the hair without focusing on the scalp to help prevent excess build up
- Make sure your shampoo and wash out conditioners are thoroughly remove
- Avoid temperature extremes by wearing a hat in cold weather, using sunscreen for hair when needed and by not applying direct heat to your scalp
- See a dermatologist or trichologist if your efforts fail to resolve your scalp issues or improve its health

Scalp Analysis Worksheet:

	Yes	No
Dandruff		
Ectoparasites		
Sores		
Alopecia		
Soreness		
Build up		

OH POO!

Who knew there were so many ways to wash your hair!

There are plenty of sites & books loaded with info about the following methods, but this will give you a brief overview so you can begin to determine which method works best for your hair!

PRE-POO: Coating the hair with conditioner or oils prior to placing shampoo on the scalp & hair

SHAMPOO: Cleansing the hair with a shampoo that usually contains sulfates

LOW-POO or LO POO: Using a non-sulfate shampoo and in some cases one that is void of silicones

CO-POO: Mixing conditioner with shampoo prior to placing it on the scalp & hair

NO-POO: No shampoo (baking soda, ACV or conditioner can be used to replace shampoo)

CO-WASH: Cleansing the scalp & hair with conditioner instead of shampoo

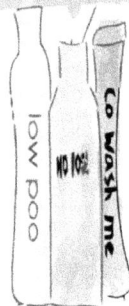

2. How does your hair feel?

When you touch your hair, does it feel dry, brittle, gummy or spongy? Get to know the texture or feel of your hair so that you can know what is normal or abnormal. Many times a lack or excess of protein can cause extremely dry or over-moisturized hair. If your hair feels too soft, some would describe this feeling as gummy or mushy, it may be an indicator of excess moisture and protein is needed. If your hair feels too dry, is brittle and breaks easily (lacks tensile strength) this could be an indicator of too much protein and moisture is needed. Of course there are many other things that can cause dry, brittle hair such as damage, too much heat and over processing.

When I touch my hair it feels? _____

I am concerned that my hair may be too _____

Did you know that the shampoo you use can affect the way your hair feels? There are several types of shampoo that produce different results!

Clarifying: These shampoos are formulated to lift and rid the hair of debris better than traditional shampoos.

Chelating: These shampoos are formulated to lift and remove deposits, including metals and minerals, from the hair that may remain with a traditional shampoo. Usually used if you have hard water.

Neutralizing: These shampoos contain a low pH used to normalize the hair's pH after a relaxer.

Moisturizing: these shampoos usually have very moisturizing properties and ingredients and are used to cleanse while replenishing moisture. Usually sulfate free.

The Natural Truth!

Understanding the difference between Natural & Organic Products is important if these are products you purchase. Not everything is what it seems, so it is important to read the ingredients listed on any product.

Natural: applies broadly to foods (or products) that are minimally processed and free of synthetic preservatives.

Organic: applies to the processing of foods (or products) & how they are produced. These items are certified under the NOP and must be grown and processed using organic methods.

After NOP certification, the products are broken into 4 categories

1. 100% organic: containing only organically produced ingredients
2. Organic: containing at least 95% organically produced ingredients
3. Made with organic ingredients: containing at least 70% organic ingredients
4. Less than 70% cannot use the word organic on the label, but may specify which ingredients are certified organic

3. Hair Products

What you put on your hair is just as important as what you put in your body. Some of these products not only affect your hair, but can negatively affect your health as well. There are so many products with varying ingredients that it can be a daunting task just choosing what you will use. Here are some tips to help you decide what to use and what not to use:

- Avoid harmful chemicals: there are many books, articles and research papers about harsh chemicals to avoid. You can use the following chart to make a list of the most prominent ones and avoid them at all cost

- Know the pH of your products: we are aware that pH affects hair, therefore knowing your product pH should be an integral part of your hair care regimen, as a general rule
  - Low pH: closes cuticles and causes slight swelling
  - High pH: opens cuticles and causes excessive swelling, this can sometimes cause breakage
- Use products as directed

- Keep a record of what was beneficial for your hair and what did not work that well

- Confer with others, although you have to ultimately decide what works for your hair getting advice from others may help you along the way

Prominent Chemicals to avoid

Tried & True (Products that I like)	Tired & Through (Products that I don't like)
✿✿✿✿✿	✿✿✿✿✿
✿✿✿✿✿	✿✿✿✿✿
✿✿✿✿✿	✿✿✿✿✿
✿✿✿✿✿	✿✿✿✿✿
✿✿✿✿✿	✿✿✿✿✿
✿✿✿✿✿	✿✿✿✿✿
✿✿✿✿✿	✿✿✿✿✿
✿✿✿✿✿	✿✿✿✿✿

A quick and easy way to keep track of products you use!

Afro Rating System!

Tried & True (Products that I like)	Tired & Through (Products that I don't like)

FAVORITE PRODUCTS

Shampoo	Conditioner	Moisturizer	Other

Getting your pH(d)

What is pH? pH stands for the potential of hydrogen and refers to the degree of acidity or alkalinity in a liquid.

What is the pH scale? The pH scale is used to measure the pH of certain liquids. It goes from 0-14 with a neutral of 7 (water). A liquid below 7 is an acid (acidic) and anything about 7 is an alkaline (basic)

What does this mean for my hair? Normal, healthy, pH balanced hair is mildly acidic (5-5.5) and optimally it will be retained within this range. It is important to know the pH of certain products used so that the pH of your hair can be maintained within its normal range. For example, may soap-based shampoos are alkaline and if used on the hair a mildly acidic rinse or product can be used after shampooing to restore pH balance.

How can I test the pH of products? pH strips are everywhere (just about) and can be purchased on-line and in many stores for a reasonable price.

The following are reference ranges for common solutions used in the hair. Bleach is included as a reference for alkalinity and should NEVER be used in the hair or on the skin. Dilutions may vary, so it is important to test the pH for yourself before placing products in the hair or on the skin and always consult your physician prior to use.

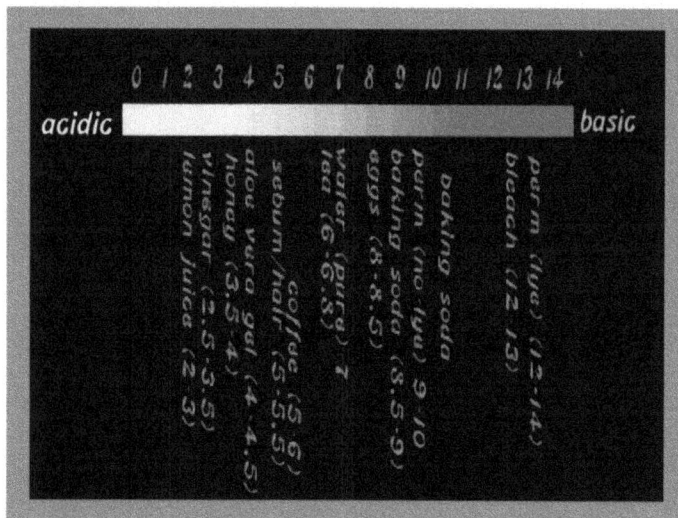

0 1 2 3 4 5 6 7 8 9 10 11 12 13 14

acidic | basic

lemon juice (2-3)
vinegar (2.5-3.5)
honey (3.5-4)
aloe vera gel (4-4.5)
sebum/hair (5-5.5)
coffee (5-6)
water (pure) 7
tea (6-6.8)
eggs (8-8.5)
baking soda (8.5-9)
perm (no lye) 9-10
baking soda
perm (lye) (12-14)
bleach (12-13)

Use the chart below to keep track of your products pH:

Shampoo	pH	Conditioner	pH	Moisturizer	pH

4. Shaft Quality

When you look at the shaft of your hair does it appear healthy? Are there splits at the end or going up the shaft? Are there tiny raised areas or 'bubbles' along the shaft which may turn into longitudinal ruptures? Are there knots present?

Knowing the condition of your hair shaft is imperative to understanding if what you have been doing is helping or hurting. Damage to the hair shaft is one of the main reasons people see breakage and why they feel that their hair will not or cannot grow! Your hair is always growing, but it could be breaking off just as quickly. Many times the only way to rid your hair of damage such as split ends, bubble hair or knots is by cutting away the offending pieces.

Notes:

_____

_____

_____

_____

_____

_____

_____

_____

_____

_____

_____

Things to avoid:

- Excessive heat: this can be very drying to the hair and scalp

- Harsh manipulation: especially when brushing and combing

- Not keeping your ends clipped as needed

- Exposing your hair to harsh environmental factors: an excess of chlorine, heat, cold and solar radiation can all cause damage to your precious strands

- Not cleansing on a regular basis: no matter how you choose to wash or cleanse your hair it should be done regularly to prevent unwanted build-up on your strands

- Excessive friction: try sleeping with a silk or satin scarf or pillow case which usually is not as harsh on the hair

- Traction: don't pull hair back too tight and try not to place a pony tail or puff in the same place too often

- Poor health: take care of your body by eating healthy foods and getting enough water

- Not getting enough sleep: sleep is a time your body uses to recharge and is needed for healthy hair and skin

- Over processing: avoid leaving treatments on for longer periods than directed

- Harsh chemicals: check the ingredients of everything you put on your hair and in your body to avoid unwanted chemicals

- Not detangling hair: this can lead to tangles, knots and frustration, therefore take the time to regularly detangle your hair

- Not being gentle with your hair: since your hair is very delicate try to be as gentle as possible when working with it

5. Hair Character

Characterizing your hair can be an important part of knowing where your strands stand. Hair characteristics vary from person to person or from strand to strand on one head of hair. The popular methods we describe here are fun to perform, but not all are scientifically proven. Many are currently used in hair salons and cosmetology schools. Of course, the best method is seeking the assistance of a professional to have your hair analyzed.

Strand thickness

The circumference of your hair strands can change due to weather, age or proximity to the scalp. It can be placed into one of three categories and one common way to determine your hair's strand thickness is by testing the way it falls.

- Fine : falls limp and flat, usually difficult to see and feel
- Medium : falls, but does not lay flat and remains lifted away from the scalp
- Thick : doesn't readily fall and will sometimes stick straight up, can feel and see the strand easily

I believe my hairs strand thickness is: _____

Density

The number of strands per one square inch, although there are many categories of hair density, we will keep it simple and divide it into three main sections. Determining your hairs density is no perfect science, but one easy way is by securing it in a hair band and measuring the circumference of your pony tail. Of course this depends on the size of the pony tail and how tightly you wrap your hair and for optimal effectiveness you want your hair as smooth as possible. Another way to determine your hairs density is by having the number of strands per square inch counted.

- Thin: a pony tail of less than two inches
- Medium: 2-3 inches
- Thick: 4 inches or more

Another popular method of determining your hair's density is by the drying time:

An hour or under: thin

Over an hour: medium

Over two hours: thick

I believe my hairs density is: _____

Elasticity

Testing the elasticity or springiness is important because it is also an indicator of hair health. The definition of elasticity is 'the ability of a strained body to recover its size and shape after deformation'. Elasticity increases when your hair is wet and can stretch a great deal!

Excessive elasticity: stretches too much and does not easily return to its original state (excess moisture)

Normal elasticity: stretches the optimal amount and easily returns to its original state

Decreased elasticity: does not stretch at all prior to breaking (decreased moisture/excess protein)

I believe my hair has: _____

Tensile Strength

Tensile strength goes hand in hand with elasticity. The definition of tensile strength is 'the greatest longitudinal stress a substance can bear without tearing apart'. The tensile strength of hair is measured by the force needed to break a strand of hair and it reduces when hair is wet. This is why it's so important to be gentle with hair in this state. If your hair is dry and brittle the tensile strength will be very low and the shaft will fracture easily.

It is said that the tensile strength of a healthy hair is approximately the same as that of a copper wire similar in size. But even if your hair is healthy and has good tensile strength it can easily be broken if sudden force is applied, therefore it is important to be gentle when combing, brushing and detangling hair.

☐ My hair breaks easily when force is applied (ends of a strand are pulled apart)

☐ My hair does not break easily when force is applied

Notes:

_____

_____

_____

_____

_____

_____

_____

Porosity

Porosity means being permeable to fluids. Determining your hairs porosity is essential when deciding the types of products you will use on your hair. The porosity of the hair depends upon the condition of the cuticle. If the cuticle is extremely porous liquids can easily pass through the cuticle scales.

Since hair porosity is extremely important and yet one of the least understood issues in hair care, we wanted to give a simple example! Think of 3 flowers, one is tightly closed, the second is opening and the third is in full bloom. Now it rains, which one do you think will get more water inside the petals? The flower in full bloom will get more rain and for our purpose will denote high porosity.

Porosity can be divided into three categories

- High: Cuticles are open and allow for water take-up and swelling (also loses moisture easily); hair is easily processed and takes color easily due to high porosity
- Normal : this is optimal, where the cuticles will allow some penetration of liquids and products, but not an excessive amount
- Low: Cuticles are tightly closed and firmly packed against each other, hair is difficult to process and color due to low porosity

How can you determine the porosity of your hair? There have been many methods described.

1. The sink or swim method: Take a strand of clean hair and place it into a cup of water, if after two minutes it sinks your hair has high porosity (taking up too much water).
2. The tactile method: still used in some cosmetology schools, is done by sliding your fingers down the length of your hair. It is said that if your hair ruffles, feels rough or

you feel bumps, your hair is porous and if it is normal your fingers will gently slide down the length of the hair shaft

There are many reasons for high porosity in hair, here are a few:

- Chemicals including relaxers, bleaching and coloring the hair have been shown to increase porosity
- Heat damage
- Chlorine
- Sun damage or UV damage

I believe my hair has _____ porosity.

Environmental factors

The environment affects your hair just as much as what you put in it. Many times these are factors that cannot be controlled, so you will have to learn to work around them to protect your hair.

- Smog, dust and other particles accumulate on your hair and contribute to build up on the hair shaft and your scalp, therefore regular clarification and cleansing are beneficial to the hair
- Sun light, UV or solar rays can negatively affect your hair, use hair products with UV protection, or cover your head with a hat when staying in the sun for long periods of time
- If you live in a very cold climate try to protect your hair. Many times the only way to do this is to make sure your ends are well covered by a protective hair style or hat. If the hat is wool or cotton, it is recommended that you place a silk or satin scarf on first to prevent excess friction

- If you are an avid swimmer make sure all the chlorine is out of your hair after leaving the pool. Covering your hair with a swim cap and applying protection can greatly reduce the damage caused by chlorine

- Humidity can be good for hair if moisture is needed, with increased humidity the hair shaft may swell allowing water to penetrate the hair shaft. You can take advantage of this by using products called humectants, such as honey and vegetable glycerin

Braving the Tight Rope!

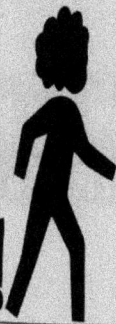

Understanding the delicate balance between protein and moisture is a necessary part of achieving healthy hair. Moisture and protein are both vital to the health of your hair, but too much of either one can cause breakage.

1. Too much protein (lacks elasticity): the hair generally feels rough, brittle and breaks easily.

2. Too much moisture (lacks structure): the hair generally feels gummy and seems to stretch for miles before it breaks.

Overmoisturizing most commonly occurs when overconditioning with products that have no protein in the ingredients. Too much protein usually occurs with sole use of products that contain protein.

Remember to read the ingredients in every product before you make a purchase to know exactly what you are putting on your hair. You are looking for ingredients that are not only healthy or safe, but also to determine if they are predominately protein building or moisturizing. Both over moisturizing and too much protein can cause damage to your tresses. It is a fine balancing act that many of us must learn, but once you do, your hair will thank you for braving the tight rope! No one can tell you the correct balance for your hair, so have patience and take notes on how your hair reacts to certain products.

You can use this as a reference for products you use.
Determine if they are high in protein (p) or mainly for moisture (m)!

Name	Notes	P	M

The condition of your hair

There has been much debate about the beneficial effects of deep conditioning treatments. But regardless of opinions, the fact remains that the application of conditioner after shampooing the hair is a necessary part of keeping your hair healthy.

One of the most important roles conditioners play in the health of our hair is balancing the pH, which by now we know is an essential aspect of healthy hair. It also serves to close the cuticles along the hair shaft and give your hair great 'slippage' for easy combing and detangling.

Deep conditioning is when heat is applied to the hair for 15 minutes or more or when the conditioner is allowed to stay on the hair for much longer periods of time. Whether this is absolutely necessary requires further research, but in the mean time, it's important to listen to your own hair so that you can decide if it will be an integral part of your regimen.

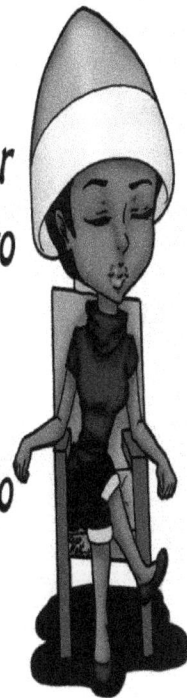

Making your regimen

Let go of your leash, take the shackles off your feet. I guarantee you'll be free and happier! Live happier. Be natural!

Fertile Ground

How you take care of your hair is one of the most important factors in your hairs health, strength, length retention & growth. For every successful endeavor, there should be a well thought out plan.

What's your plan for your hair? Map it out thoroughly & stick with it!

If your routine or regimen works for you three months from now, continue with it. If not change it up a bit until you find out what works for your hair.

Please refer to the Happy Hair Glossary for the definitions of abbreviated terms

Making your Regimen

When considering a regimen there are many questions to ask yourself before you start.

How often will I wash my hair?

What products will I use & on what schedule

Will I deep condition?

What styles will I use?

Who will clip my ends?

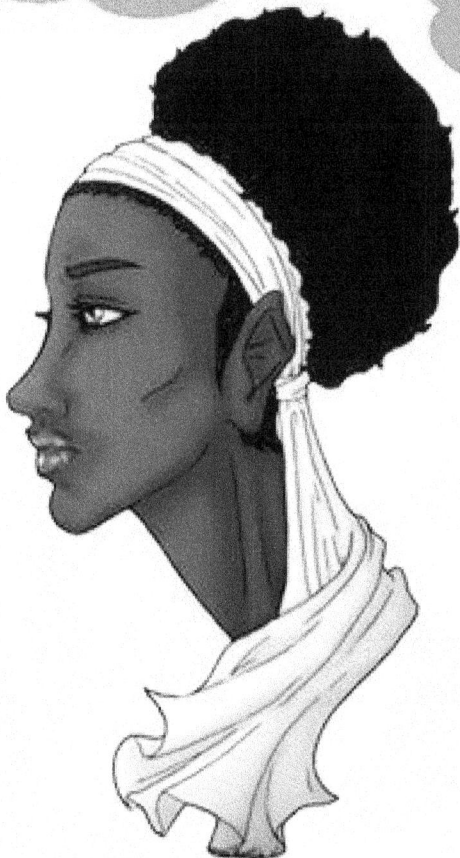

Other Questions you may want to consider when making your regimen:

- How will I wash my hair?
- How much water will I drink per day?
- What protective styles will I use?
- What products will I use?
- Will I go to the salon and how often?
- When will I deep condition?
- How often will I clip my ends?
- How will I clip my ends?
- Will I use protein treatments?
- Will I co-wash or use shampoo?
- What type of shampoo will I use (sulfate free/with sulfates)?
- How often will I wet my hair?
- Will I baggy my hair and if so how often?
- Will I need a water softener when washing my hair?
- How often will I clarify?
- Will I need to use a chelating shampoo?
- Which of my conditioners have proteins?
- What is the length of my hair currently?
- What are my overall goals for my hair?
- What are my short-term goals for my hair?
- What are my long-term goals for my hair?
- My personal mental shift goal is?

MY HAIR REGIMEN

DAILY

NIGHTLY

WEEKLY

EVERY OTHER WEEK

MONTHLY

EVERY 3 MONTHS

Length check:_____ Date:_____

My hair goals for the next 3 months

My Natural Hair Journey

Date taken:

What I have learned about my hair thus far

Likes

Dislikes

Getting to know you question:
How many textures do I have?

3 months

MY HAIR REGIMEN

DAILY

NIGHTLY

WEEKLY

EVERY OTHER WEEK

MONTHLY

EVERY 3 MONTHS

Length check:_____ Date:_____

My hair goals for the next 3 months

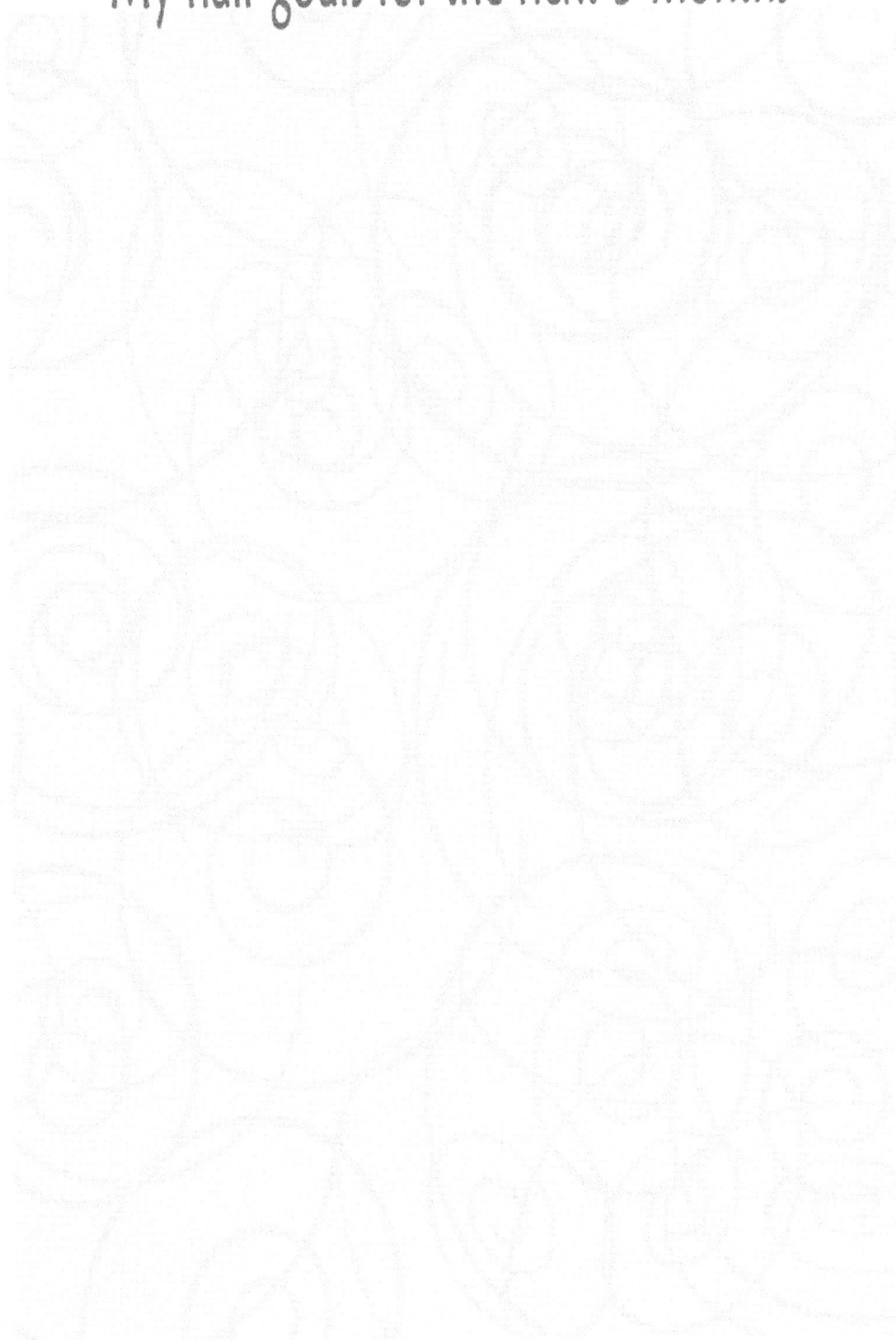

My Natural Hair Journey

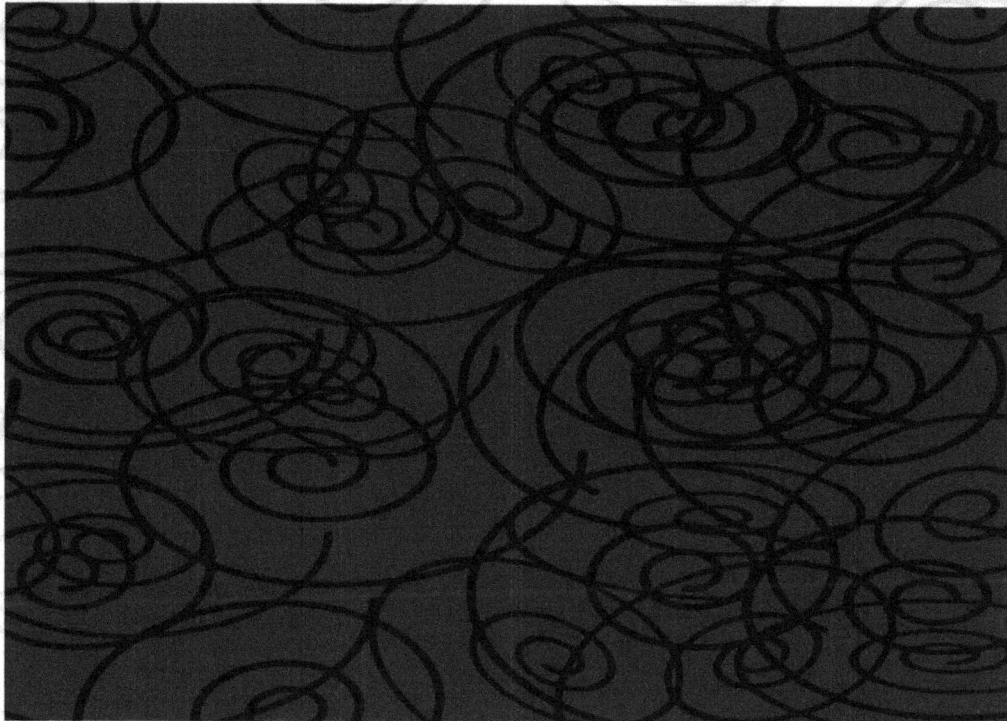

Date taken:

What I have learned about my hair thus far

Likes

Dislikes

Getting to know you question:
About how much shedding is normal
for my hair when detangling?

6 months

MY HAIR REGIMEN

DAILY

NIGHTLY

WEEKLY

EVERY OTHER WEEK

MONTHLY

EVERY 3 MONTHS

Length check:_____ Date:_____

My hair goals for the next 3 months

My Natural Hair Journey

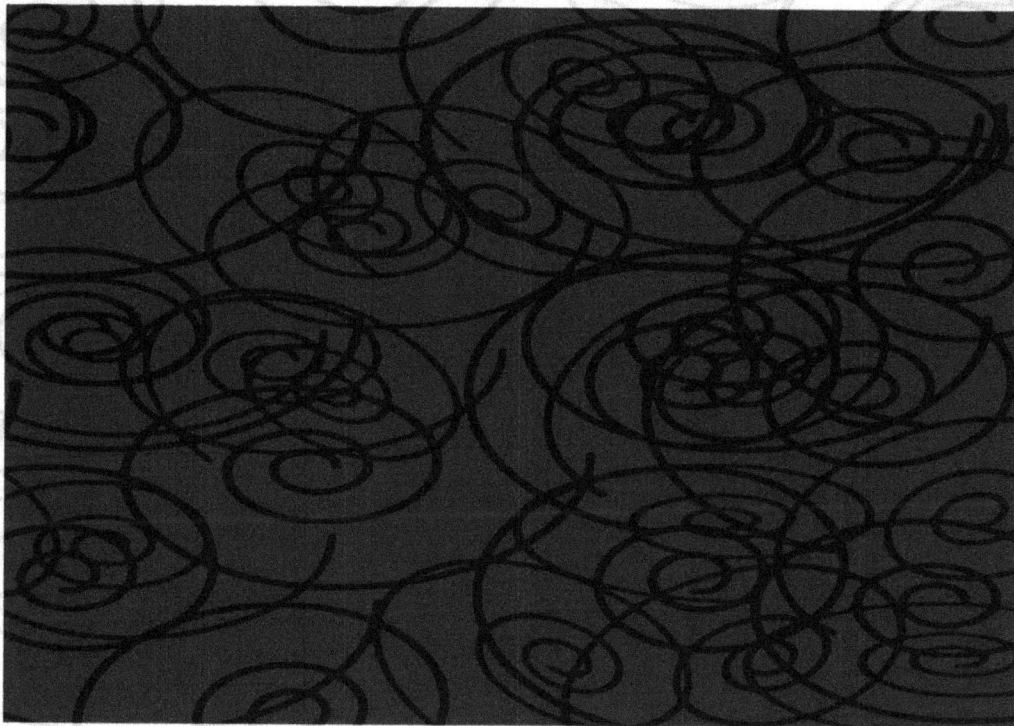

Date taken:

What I have learned about my hair thus far

Likes

Dislikes

Getting to know you question
How many inches does my hair
grow a month?

_____

9 months

MY HAIR REGIMEN

DAILY

NIGHTLY

WEEKLY

EVERY OTHER WEEK

MONTHLY

EVERY 3 MONTHS

Length check:_____ Date:_____

My hair goals for the next 3 months

My Natural Hair Journey

Date taken:

What I have learned about my hair thus far

Likes

Dislikes

Getting to know you question
What part of my hair grows the fastest?

BACK ■　　FRONT ■　　SIDES ■　　MIDDLE ■

12 months

Length Check

Date				
	Length	Length	Length	Length
Front				
Middle				
Right Side				
Left Side				
Right Back				
Left Back				
Middle Back				

Hair Recipes I love

Name

Ingredients

Name

Ingredients

Hair Recipes I love

Name

Ingredients

Name

Ingredients

Hair Recipes I love

Name

Ingredients

Name

Ingredients

Hair Recipes I love

Name

Ingredients

Name

Ingredients

Protective Challenge

Protective challenges have been toted as a great way to retain length by keeping your ends well moisturized and hidden away from external influences. They can be found all over the internet or you can choose to do one with your friends!

Participants

Length of time

My hair stats start

My hair stats end

Rules

Protective Challenge

Protective challenges have been toted as a great way to retain length by keeping your ends well moisturized and hidden away from external influences. They can be found all over the internet or you can choose to do one with your friends!

Participants

Length of time

My hair stats start

My hair stats end

Rules

Protective Challenge

Protective challenges have been toted as a great way to retain length by keeping your ends well moisturized and hidden away from external influences. They can be found all over the internet or you can choose to do one with your friends!

Participants

Length of time

My hair stats start

My hair stats end

Rules

Protective Challenge

Protective challenges have been toted as a great way to retain length by keeping your ends well moisturized and hidden away from external influences. They can be found all over the internet or you can choose to do one with your friends!

Participants

Length of time

My hair stats start

My hair stats end

Rules

Favorite Video Personalities

Favorite Blogs

Upcoming Hair Events

Not what the main stream image is,
natural hair is your heritage but to see
it without chemicals is rare as the
pyramids
Dead Prez

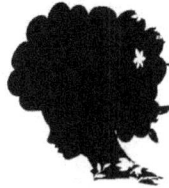

The world of hair has grown tremendously over the past couple of years especially the natural hair world. As expected, the vocabulary used on many websites and blogs has increased exponentially as well. The following is a comprehensive glossary of common acronyms, abbreviations and terminology used in the hair world and on hair forums. Some terms and abbreviations may have several meanings, but we have focused on the consensual usage as it pertains to hair.

Please use any products mentioned in the glossary or in the text of this book only after consulting your primary care physician.

Happy Hair Glossary

A

ABS: African Black Soap

Accordion method: A technique used to enhance curl definition by gently pressing wet hair coated with product toward the scalp from tip to root

A-cone: amodimethicone (a silicone)

ACV: Apple Cider Vinegar

Afro: Curly hair that has been picked out and shaped into a round style around the head

Alopecia: The loss of hair

ALS: Ammonium Lauryl Sulfates

ALES: Ammonium Laureth Sulfates

APL: Arm Pit Length

AV: 1.Aloe Vera 2. American Vendor

AVG: Aloe Vera Gel

AVJ: Aloe Vera Juice

AVI: Avatar, small pictures used in most hair care forums

B

BA: Big Afro (An afro that is 8-12 inches in length)

BAA: Bad Ass Afro or Big Ass Afro (An afro that is over 12 inches in length)

Backcombing: Combing the hair toward the scalp to ensure knotting. This process is commonly used to start locks (dreadlocks) on hair that is too straight to curl or twist around itself

Banding Method: Stretching hair by applying numerous rubber bands, 'scrunchies' or other hair accessory along the length of the hair in an effort to revert or prevent shrinkage usually during the drying processes

Baggy (Baggying or Baggy Method): A method where a moisture based product is applied and hair is covered with a plastic bag or cap and secured with a scarf if desired. Oil can be applied after removal of the cap to seal in moisture

Bantu Knot: Hair is sectioned into small areas, held at the root with one hand close the scalp and twisted around itself in a circular motion until it forms what resembles a knot. Once there is a small piece of hair left it is usually tucked under the knot close to the scalp. Also known as Zulu knots

Bantu Knot Out: Removal of Bantu Knots and wearing the hair in a curly style

Beeswax: The wax secreted by honeybees for constructing honeycombs, many times it is used to start or maintain locks (dreadlocks)

Bentonite: A type of clay sometimes used as a purifying hair mask

BBB: 1. Boar Bristle Brush; 2. Better Business Bureau

BC: big chop or big cut, cutting away permed or relaxed hair to have all natural hair

Blow Out: Blow-drying the hair section by section until it is straight. It also refers to a hair style

BNC: Braid and Curl, the hair is braided and the ends are curled usually using rollers, rods or curling iron

Box Braids: Individual braids that are not close to the scalp

Bubble hair: an irreversible acquired shaft deformity seen microscopically that is said to be precipitated by using excessive heat

Buds (Budding): Short twist, the initial stage of locking the hair

Build-up: Dirt, debris and residue left by products placed in hair, this can prevent much needed moisture & beneficial oils from penetrating the hair shaft

BUMP: Bring Up My Post, abbreviation commonly used on forums to keep a post at the forefront

BSL: Bra Strap Length

BSS: Beauty Supply Store

C

C: Describes a coarse texture of hair

Canopy: The top layer of hair, it is exposed to the elements the most

CB: Curly butter

CBL: collar bone length

CD: Curl definition

CG: Curly Girl

Chelating Shampoo: A shampoo used to remove deposits, including metal ions and minerals that a clarifying shampoo may miss

CL: Chin Length

Clarifying Shampoo: A shampoo used specifically to remove deposits (oil, build-up) from the hair

Clumping: When smaller sections or strands of hair stick together and form large sections of hair

CO: 1. Castor oil 2. Coconut oil 3. Conditioner 4. Conditioner only

Co-add or co-a: conditioner additive, a product (usually an oil or butter) added to a conditioner

Combination hair: Having more than one pattern or texture of hair on one's head

Comb Coils: A process commonly used to begin locks (dreadlocks) where a small section of hair is gently twisted around a rattail comb to create a coil pattern

Condish: Conditioner

Conditioner washing: Co-washing

Co-poo: Mixing conditioner with shampoo prior to applying to the hair

Co-wash: Cleansing hair using only conditioner (no shampoo is used)

Cones: Refers to silicones in hair products

Cornrow: a style where the hair is braided very close to the scalp in a continuous motion

CP: 1. Curly pudding 2. Curl pudding

Creamy Crack: 1. Perm 2. Relaxer 3. Chemical processing of the hair

Crunch: See crunchy

Crunchy: When a product (usually one of gel consistency) leaves hair feeling brittle and hard to the touch, the hair may make a 'crunching' sound when touched. As the product dries flakes may form on the hair and scalp

Cultivated locks: Locks that are parted and maintained for uniformity by tightening each section on a regular basis, these locks are usually around the same size, length and shape

Curl Definition: When individual strands of hair come together to form a distinctive curl pattern

CW: Conditioner wash (co-wash)

CWC: condition-wash-condition routine

D

DC: Deep conditioning or Deep conditioner

DCT: Deep conditioning treatment

Diffuser: An attachment that comes with most hair dryers, it is used to dry the hair using low air flow, sometimes used to give the hair lift and often used so the curl pattern is not interrupted while drying

D.I.Y: Do it yourself

DL: Dreadlocks

DMDM–Hydantoin: a formaldehyde releasing chemical used in some beauty products

DPT: Deep protein treatment

Dreadlock wax: usually a mixture of beeswax & other oils or a wax alternative used to start or continue locks (dreadlocks) by helping the hair stick together

DT: Deep Treatment (conditioner)

Dusting: Trimming a small amount from the ends of the hair. Usually about $1/4^{th}$ -$1/12^{th}$ of an inch or less

E

EFA: Essential Fatty Acids

EL: Ear Length

EO: Essential Oils

EPO: Evening Primrose Oil

ETA: Edited to add, commonly used on forums

EVCO: Extra Virgin Coconut Oil

EVOO: Extra Virgin Olive Oil

∞◌◌

Hair produces its own protective oil called sebum. Sebum is actually secreted from most areas of the skin by sebaceous glands.

∞◌◌

F

F: describes a fine texture of hair

Fairy knots: Also known as single strand knots, these are knots found on single strands of hair and named so because of their small size

Finger combing: Using the fingers to comb the hair

Finger Twist: A method commonly used to start locks (dreadlocks) where sections of hair are gently twisted around the finger into a coil like pattern

Flat twist: Taking two sections of hair and twisting them in a continuous motion very close to the scalp, similar to a cornrow

Fluffing: The process of using the fingertips to lightly lift hair away from the scalp, it is done to achieve maximum volume

FO: Fragrance oils

Freeform locks: Hair is pulled together in clusters or large sections after each wash without regard to uniformity, these locks usually come in various sizes, locks are washed for maintenance but very little else is done to tighten or maintain them

FSG: Flax Seed Gel

G

GHE: Green House Effect

GLY: Glycerin

GOC: Grow Out Challenge

Good Hair: See the hair on top of your head

Greenhouse effect: Method similar to the Baggy method where natural oils are used instead of a moisturizing base. The oils are allowed to coat the hair shaft, a plastic bag or shower cap is placed on the head and secured with a scarf if desired. Usually done overnight, the body generates heat and moisture

GSO: Grape Seed Oil

ॐ

Once hair is damaged there is very little that can be done to repair it.

ॐ

H

Hair Density: The number of individual hair strands per square inch or a given area

Hair Follicle Density: The density of hair follicle structures in the skin

Hair Regimen: A schedule followed consistently for hair care

Hard Water: Water that contains a high mineral content

HCF: Hair care forum

HD: Heat damage

Heat Training: The use of consistent heat over a period of time to straighten naturally curly, kinky or coily hair in an effort to discourage reversion

Henna: A flowering plant used to dye skin, hair, nails and other things

HFS: Health food store

HG: Holy Grail, products and routines that are used consistently in a regimen

HH: Human Hair

HHG: 1. Happy Hair Growing 2. Happy Hair Growth 3. Healthy Hair Growth

HHJ: 1. Healthy Hair Journey 2. Happy Hair Journey

HIA: Hand in afro; a 'disease' where one is obsessed with their afro and cannot keep their hands out of it

HIH: Hand in hair; a 'disease' where one is obsessed with their hair and unable to keep their hands out of it

HM: Homemade

HL: Hip length

H.O.T: Hot oil treatment

HT: Heat training

Humectant: A substance that attracts moisture, such as honey or vegetable glycerin

Hydrolyzed: The process of breaking down proteins into amino acids. This usually indicates a protein in the ingredients of a product

Hygral fatigue: The process of swelling and deswelling of the hair due to water use; it can cause damage to the hair which may be limited by the use of oils

I

IMHO: In my humble or honest opinion

ISO: In search of (used on forums)

J

JJ: (JjJ) Jojoba jelly

JJO: (JO) Jojoba oil

K

Keratin: A type of protein found in hair, skin and nails

KL: Knee Length

KT: Keratin Treatment

L

Lecithin: a group of phospholipids found in the cells of many plants and animals, used as an emulsifier in many commercial products and foods

LI: leave in conditioner

LIC: 1. Leave in conditioner 2. License

Line of demarcation: Occurs during the transition phase, the area on the hair where relaxed hair meets the natural hair

L.O.C: Liquid Oil Cream (method)

Locks (Dreadlocks): A style where the hair is intertwined around itself using wax or other products and maintained in the twisted or matted state by not brushing or combing the hair

Locs: dreadlocks

Loctician: (locktician) A person that specializes in starting, grooming, maintaining and trimming locks (dreadlocks) also known as dreadlock stylist

LOTD: Look of the day

Low Poo: Using a non-sulfate shampoo and in some cases silicone free as well

M

M: describes medium textured hair

MBL: Mid Back Length

೫**ෲ**

On average, hair grows at a rate of about half an inch per month

೫**ෲ**

N

Naked Hair: Hair with no product, usually freshly washed

Nappyversary: The anniversary of becoming fully natural or having hair without chemical process

NB: Nappy Birthday

NC: Naturally curly

Newbie: Someone new to the natural hair process

New Growth: The hair closest to the scalp that has recently grown since a process or style such as a relaxer or braids

NG: New Growth

NL: 1.Nape Length 2.Neck Length

NOP: National Organic Program.

No-Poo: Cleansing hair without shampoo, in some cases baking soda or ACV rinses are used in place of shampoo & in some cases conditioners are used (co-wash) to replace shampoo. This also eliminates the use of sulfates and silicones in the hair

NV: Nappyversary

NW: No water method of cleansing the hair and scalp, baking soda is commonly used for this method

O

OC: Over conditioned

OM: Over moisturized

OO: Olive oil

OP: Original Poster or Original Post, used on forums to refer to the person starting a thread

Organic locks: locks (dreadlocks) that are allowed to form without manipulation, these locks usually have a matted appearance and are various shapes and sizes

ഓരു

About 70-80% of the hair is made of keratin (protein), as well as water, melanin (pigment) and trace elements.

ഓരു

P

Palm Rolling: Method for starting and maintaining locks (dreadlocks) where the hair is rolled between the base of the palms to create a coiled pattern

PDTs: Products

pH: potential of hydrogen, the measure of acidity or alkalinity of an aqueous solution

PHHB: Panty Hose Head Band

Pineappleing: Gathering all of your hair into a high bun or ponytail on the crown of the head, secured with a ponytail holder or other hair accessory while sleeping on a satin or silk pillow case. This method is used to preserve the curl definition

Pixie Curl Diffuser Method: A method of drying hair to decrease the chance of frizz and flyaways. The hair is gathered under the diffuser and placed very close to the scalp, hair is dried like this for a minute or two. The diffuser is then turned off when moving to a different section to prevent blowing the hair. The method is repeated on the entire head until dry

PJ: product junkie, a person that continuously purchases hair products & can't stop

Plaits: Braids

Plopping: A method of drying hair with a material that is 'hair' friendly in some cases a t-shirt or micro-fiber towel (hair friendly towel) is draped over the head for a 15-20 min and removed. This method is used instead of rubbing the hair with a towel. Also known as Plunking

Plunking: see plopping

PM: Private message

Poo: Shampoo

Poo-bar: Shampoo bar

Pop: The enhancement of curl definition, usually seen after a shake-n-go or application of a product

Porosity: the ease with which the hair absorbs and retains liquid or moisture. It can range from high, normal to low

Pre-Poo: coating the hair with conditioner or oils approximately 20-30 min prior to washing with shampoo or low-poo (pre-shampoo treatment)

PS: Protective Style, a style where the hair is up and the ends of the hair are protected and not exposed to the elements. Usually these are styles that can last for days for to ensure manipulation

PT: Protein Treatments

Puff: Hair that is in an afro state gathered together with a hair accessory, usually in one or two large sections

PVP: Polyvinylpyrrolidone (polyvidone), a water soluble polymer used in many hair sprays and gels

PW: Password

Q

Quats: Polyquaternium or Poly (diallyldimethylammonium chloride) a polymer that is colorless. It is used in some conditioners, shampoos, hair sprays, dyes and other cosmetics. They can build-up on the hair shaft similar to cones

R

Relaxer: A chemical lotion or cream used to make the hair less curly or straight. 'Relaxing' natural curls. Perm

RO: Rinse out (conditioner)

Revert: When naturally curly hair that is in a straight state returns to its normal curl pattern (reversion)

S

S&D : Search and Destroy, Method of trimming hair, where split ends or knots on individual strands are found and clipped

SAO: Sweet Almond Oil

SB: Shea Butter

Scab Hair: Relaxed hair that is not removed at the time of a big chop, many times this is unintentional

Scrunch: Applying or removing excess moisture or product from the hair by pressing or squeezing firmly on curls. This is usually done in an upward motion, starting at the tip of the hair strand and pressing or squeezing towards the scalp

SD: Seborrheic dermatitis

Sealing: Preventing moisture from leaving the hair by placing a moisture based product or water on the hair and layering it with an oil or butter, usually done post washing

Sebum: The natural oil produced by skin

Second day hair: hair that remains 'wearable' the day after the style is done (2nd day hair)

Shake-n-go: After hair is wet, the head is vigorously shaken back and forth or side to side to make curls 'pop' and hair dry

Shingling: a method used to define and elongate curls by applying a cream based product, combing it through with a small tooth comb and sitting under the dryer or using a diffuser to dry

Shrinkage: A term used when curly, kinky or coily hair shortens as it dries due to the tightness of the curls

SSKS: Single strand knots, also known as Fairy knots. Small knots found on the hair shaft of individual hairs

SL: Shoulder length

SLES: Sodium lauryl ether sulfate

SLS: Sodium lauryl sulfates

Slip: When hair is easily combed or it is very easy to run your fingers through the hair. Hair is usually coated with conditioner or another product

SLS: Sodium laureth sulfates

SOTC: Scruch out the Crunch

Stretching Hair: 1.(natural hair) lengthening shrunken hair through a method such as banding or plaiting. 2. (relaxed hair) waiting for an extended period of time between perms

Stripped: 1. Describes the feeling when a shampoo removes the oils out of hair leaving the hair feeling dry 2. When color or dye has been removed from the hair

Sulf: Sulfate

Synthetic locks: lock (dreadlock) extensions

T

TA: Teeny Afro (Afro that is 4-8 inches in length)

TBC: The big chop

TBL: Tailbone length (also see TLBN)

Texlax: (texlaxing; texlaxed hair) 1. A chemical relaxer or perm that is left on the hair for a shorter amount of time (usually half the directed contact time) 2. When the strength of the usual perm is reduced to allow for a longer application process. 3. Dilution of a relaxer or perm with an oil or other product. Hair does not get 'bone' straight using this process

Texturizer: A chemical process that loosens the natural curl pattern of the hair

TCM: Tightly Curly Method

Three Strand Twist: Taking three sections or hair and wrapping them around each other (very different from braids & two-strand twist)

TLBN: Tailbone Length

TNC: Twist-N-Curl. Hair is twisted and the ends curled, usually with rollers or rods

Traditional locks: locks formed by using comb coils to begin the initial pattern and usually maintained by palm rolling. These locks fall under the umbrella of cultivated locks

TR: Thermal Reconditioning, a method of straightening curly or wavy hair using heat and chemicals to restructure the hair bonds permanently

Transition: The stage when hair is in the process of growing out of a relaxer or perm and the new growth remains unprocessed

Trim: Clipping the ends of the hair in an effort to rid the strands of knots and splits. Usually about 1-2 inches are lost during the process

TTO: Tea Tree Oil

TWA: Teeny Weeny Afro (Afro that is less than 4 inches in length)

Twist out: A style achieved by two or three strand twisting the hair until it forms a spiral pattern, then unraveling each twist.

Two-Strand Twist: Taking two sections of the hair and wrapping them around each other

U

Understory: The hair under the top or exposed hair (hair under the canopy)

V

Veggie Gly: Vegetable glycerin

VG: vegetable glycerin

W

W&G: Wash and Go

Wash and Go: Washing the hair and applying a conditioner or gel to define curls

Wet and Go: Wetting the hair with water and usually applying a leave in conditioner to define curls

WL: Waist Length

WNG: Wash and go or wet and go

WO: Water Only method, using only water to cleanse the hair and scalp

WP: 1. Wheat protein 2. Whipped Pudding

WSC: Water Soluble Cone (should not cause build-up even if a shampoo is not used)

WT: Water

WTC: Wide Tooth Comb

Wurly: Hair patterns that are a cross between waves and curls

X

XG: Xanthan Gum, a natural sugar derived from corn. Commonly used as a food thickening agent

Y

Z

ZO: Zinc Oxide

Zulu knots: See bantu knots

Today I reign in my true mane
Alison Crockett

Special thanks to the following artist for allowing us to include their inspiring words and for encouraging and promoting those that choose to rock beautiful, natural, nappy hair!

Alison Crocket – Nappy

Album: The Return of Diva Blue: On Becoming a Woman Redux

www.alisoncrockett.net

Dead Prez – The Beauty Within

Writing credit: Khnum "stic" Ibomu of dead prez

Courtesy of Boss Up Inc

www.sticrbg.com

www.rbgfitclub.com

Fertile Ground/Navasha Daya – Be Natural

Album: Spiritual War

www.blackoutstudios.com

www. http://navashadaya.com

Bibliography

1. American Academy of Dermatology 69th Annual Meeting. (2011) Going to great lengths for beautiful hair? Dermatologist shares hair care tips for healthy and damaged hair. (Feb).

2. Alander J., Anderson A. The Shea butter family-the complete emollient range for skin care formulations. http://www.sheabuttermarket.com/documents/KARLSHAMNS.pdf

3. Al-Reza S.M., Yoon J.I., Kim H.J., Kim J.S., Kang S.C. (2010) Anti-inflammatory activity of seed essential oil from *Zizyphus jujuba*. Food and Chemical Toxicology, Feb; 48(2):639-643.

4. Christian P., Winsey N., Whatmough M., Cornwell PA. (2011), The effects of water on heat-styling damage. Journal of Cosmetic Science, Jan/Feb; 62(1):15-27.

5. Crawford R., Robbins C.R. (1981), A hysteresis in heat dried hair. Journal of the Society of Cosmetic Chemists, Jan/Feb; 32: 27-36

6. Dias T. C. d. S., Baby A. R., Kaneko T. M. and Velasco M. V. R. (2008), Protective effect of conditioning agents on Afro-ethnic hair chemically treated with thioglycolate-based straightening emulsion. Journal of Cosmetic Dermatology, 7: 120–126.

7. Evans T.A., Park K. (2010), A Statistical analysis of hair breakage. II. Repeated grooming experiments. Journal of Cosmetic Science, Nov/Dec ; 61(6):439-455.

8. Food marketing Institute: Natural and Organic Foods, FMI backgrounder. www.fmi.org

9. Fregonesi A., Scanavez C., Santos L., De Oliveira A., rosier R., Esxudeiro C. Moncayo P., De Sanctis D., Gesztesi J.L. (2009), Brazilian oils and butters: the effect of different fatty acid cahin composition on human hair physiochemical properties. Journal of Cosmetic Science, March/April; 60(2):273-280.

10. Guenther E. Recent developments in the field of essential oils.

11. Hay I.C., Jamieson M., Ormerod A.D. (1998), Randomized trial of aromatherapy. Successful treatment for alopecia areata. Archives of Dermatology, Nov; 134(11):1349-1352.

12. Itin P.H., Fistarol S.K. (2005), Hair Shaft Abnormalities-Clues to Diagnosis and Treatment. Dermatology, 211: 63-71.

13. Jung K., Herrling T., Blume G., et al. (2006) Detection of UV induced free radicals in hair and their prevention by hair care products. SOFW journal 132:32-36.

14. Keis K., Persaud D., Kamath Y.K., Rele A.S. (2005), Investigation of penetration abilities of various oils into human hair fibers. Journal of Cosmetic Science, Sept/Oct; 56, 283-295

15. Kelly S.E., Robinson V.N.E. (1982), The effect of grooming on the hair cuticle. Journal of the Society of Cosmetic Chemists, July; 33:203-215.

16. Lacharriere O Deloche C. et al (2011), A clinical sign reflecting the follicle miniaturization. Arch Dermatology, May; 137: 641-647

17. Massey L., Bender M. (2011), Curly Girl: The handbook. Finding your curl type, (19-27)

18. McMichael A.J. (2007), Hair breakage in normal and weathered hair: focus on the Black patient. Journal of Investigative Dermatology, Dec; 12(2): 6-9.

19. McMullen R., Jachowicz J. (1998). Thermal degradation of hair. II. Effect of selected polymers and surfactants. Journal of Cosmetic Science, July/Aug; 49:245-256.

20. Merriam-Webster's Collegiate Dictionary.

21. Mhaskar S., Kalghatgi B. Chavan M. Rout S. Gode V. (2011). Hair breakage index: An alternative tool for damage assessment of human hair. Journal of Cosmetic Science, Mar/Apr; 62 (2):203-207.

22. Moghtader M., Afzali D. (2009). Study of the antimicrobial properties of the essential oil of rosemary. American –Eurasian Journal of Agricultural and Environmental Sciences, 5(3)393-397.

23. Parker L. Hair loss and grey hair prevention with a healthy diet. American Hair Growth Centers Journal, (August 2008) www.americanhairgrowthjournal.com

24. R.D Sinclair. Doctor's resource on Bubble Hair, (May 2000).

25. Reich C., Robbins C.R. (1993). Interactions of cationic and anionic surfactants on hair surfaces: Light-scattering and radiotracer studies. Journal of the Society of Cosmetic Chemists, Sept/Oct; 44: 263-278.

26. Rele A.S., Mohile R.B. (1999), Effect of coconut oil on prevention of hair damage. Part I. Journal of Cosmetic Science, Nov/Dec; 50:327-339.

27. Rele A.S., Mohile R.B. (2003), Effect of mineral oil, sunflower oil, and coconut oil on prevention of hair damage. Journal of Cosmetic Science, March/April; 54:175-192.

28. Rigoletto R., Zhou Y., Foltis L. (2007), Semi-permanent split end mending with a polyelectrolyte complex. Journal of Cosmetic Science, July/Aug; 58:451-476.

29. Robbins C. (2006), Hair breakage during combing. I. Pathways of breakage. Journal of Cosmetic Science, May/June; 57:233-243.

30. Robbins C., Kamath Y. (2007), Hair breakage during combing. III. The effects of bleaching and conditioning on short and long segment breakage by wet and dry combing of tresses. Journal of Cosmetic Science, July/Aug; 58: 477-484.

31. Robbins C., Kamath Y. (2007), Hair breakage during combing. IV. Brushing and combing hair. Journal of Cosmetic Science; 58:629-636.

32. Robinson V.N.E. (1976), A study of damaged hair. Journal of the Society of Cosmetic Chemists. 27: 155-161.

33. Rucker Wright D., Gathers R. Kapke A., Johnson D. Joseph C.L. (2011), Hair care practices and their association with scalp and hair disorders in African American girls. Journal of the American Academy of Dermatology. Feb; 64(2): 253-62.

34. Ruetsch S.B., Kamath Y.K, Kintrup L., Schwark H.J. (2003), Effects of conditioners on surface hardness of hair fibers: an investigation using atomic force microscopy. Nov/Dec; 546):579-588.

35. Ruetsch S.B., Kamath Y.K., Rele A.S. Mohile R.B. (2001), Secondary ion mass spectrometric investigation of penetration of coconut and mineral oils into human hair fibers: Relevance to hair damage. Journal of Cosmetic Science. May/June; 52:169-184.

36. Ruetsch S.B., Kamath Y.K. (2004), Effects of thermal treatments with a curling iron on hair fiber. Journal of Cosmetic Science, Jan/Feb; 55(1): 13-27

37. Sapion S. Carlotti M.E., Peira E., Gallarate M. (2005), Hemp-seed and olive oils: Their stability against oxidation and use in O/W emulsions. Journal of Cosmetic Science; July/Aug; 56:227-251.

38. Sandhu S.S., Ramachandran R., Robbins C.R. (1995), A simple and sensitive method using protein loss measurements to evaluate damage to human hair during combing. Journal of the Society of Cosmetic Chemists , Jan/Feb; 46:39-52.

39. Syed A., Ayoub H. (2002) Correlating porosity and tensile strength of chemically modified hair. Cosmetics and toiletries magazine. November; 117: 57-64

40. Swift J.A. (1997), Mechanism of split-end formation in human head hair, Journal of the Society of Cosmetic Chemists, March/April; 48:123-126.

41. Tate M.L., Kamath Y.K., Ruetsch S.B., Weigmann H.D. (1993), Quantification and prevention of hair damage. Journal of the Society of Cosmetic Chemists, Nov/Dec; 44:347-371.

42. United States Department of Agriculture Agricultural Marketing Service. Cosmetics, body care products, and personal care products. (April 2008). www.ams.usda.gov/nop

43. Walker A., Wiltz T. (1998), Andre talks hair

44. Yoon J.I., Al-Reza S.M., Kang S.C. (2010), Hair growth promoting effect of *Zizyphus jujuba* essential oil. Food and Chemical Toxicology, Feb; 48:1350-1354.

www.ingramcontent.com/pod-product-compliance
Lightning Source LLC
Chambersburg PA
CBHW081658270326
41933CB00017B/3213